AuthorHouse™
1663 Liberty Drive
Bloomington, IN 47403
www.authorhouse.com
Phone: 1 (800) 839-8640

Published by AuthorHouse 05/04/2018

ISBN: 978-1-5462-3930-7 (sc)
978-1-5462-3931-4 (e)

Library of Congress Control Number: 2018905147

Print information available on the last page.

Any people depicted in stock imagery provided by Getty Images are models,
and such images are being used for illustrative purposes only.
Certain stock imagery © Getty Images.

This book is printed on acid-free paper.

authorHOUSE®

Mobility Exercises

Exercises to Relieve Pain, Decrease Risk of Injury, Increase Range of Motion, Improve Your Stability and Posture

JASON DOWNIE

Table of Contents

Dedication

I dedicate this book to those who believe in themselves and never give up on life.

The Human Muscular System

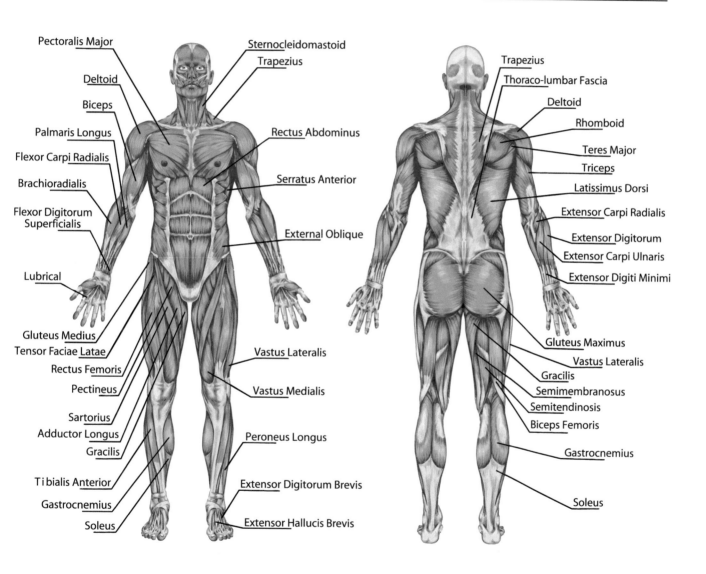

Pectoralis Major
Sternocleidomastoid
Trapezius
Deltoid
Biceps
Palmaris Longus
Rectus Abdominus
Flexor Carpi Radialis
Brachioradialis
Serratus Anterior
Flexor Digitorum Superficialis
External Oblique
Lubrical
Gluteus Medius
Tensor Faciae Latae
Rectus Femoris
Vastus Lateralis
Pectineus
Vastus Medialis
Sartorius
Adductor Longus
Gracilis
Peroneus Longus
Tibialis Anterior
Extensor Digitorum Brevis
Gastrocnemius
Soleus
Extensor Hallucis Brevis

Trapezius
Thoraco-lumbar Fascia
Deltoid
Rhomboid
Teres Major
Triceps
Latissimus Dorsi
Extensor Carpi Radialis
Extensor Digitorum
Extensor Carpi Ulnaris
Extensor Digiti Minimi
Gluteus Maximus
Vastus Lateralis
Gracilis
Semimembranosus
Semitendinosis
Biceps Femoris
Gastrocnemius
Soleus

Foam Roller and Exercises

Foam Roller

There are several mobility tools you can use to release muscle tightness. Foam rollers are a popular tool for self-myofascial release and self-massage. You can use a foam roller to treat your glutes, hamstrings, quads, back and lats. Foam rolling can be done before or after a workout. They come in different sizes and densities, so make sure you pick one that is right for you.

Gluteus Muscles (Glutes)

Too much sitting can cause your gluteus muscles to tighten up. A tight gluteus can limit your range of motion, cause poor balance, pain in the back, hips, hamstrings and other areas.

Gluteus Roll

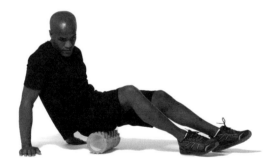 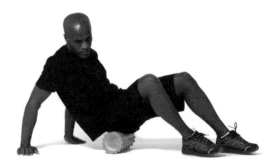

Sit on the broad side of the foam roller and place your hands on the floor behind you for support. Roll your glutes back and forth over the roller. Roll for 2-3 minutes.

Quadriceps Femoris (Quads)

Our quadriceps can tighten up from being physical active, and sitting for long periods of time. Tight quads can affect our performance, posture, the blood flow in our legs and cause lower back and knee pain.

Quadricep Roll

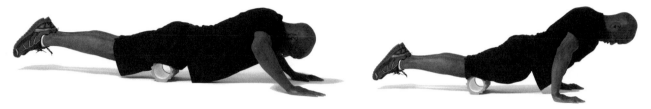

Get in a press up position with the front of both thighs on the foam roller. Roll from the top of your hips to the top of your knee caps and back to the starting position. Roll for 2-3 minutes.

Hamstring

Your hamstrings can tighten up if we were born with natural short hamstrings and if you have an anterior pelvic tilt. Not enough stretching can also cause your hamstrings to tighten up.

Hamstring Roll

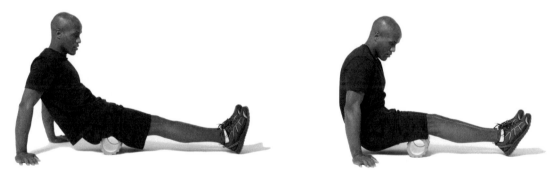

Place the foam roller under the back of your thighs and place your hands on the floor behind you to support your weight. Roll from your glutes to the back of your knees and back to the starting position. Roll for 2-3 minutes.

Groin

Have you ever felt pain in your groin while exercising? You may have tight hip adductors or a weak gluteus medius. It's possible not to know that your groin is tight until you get injured.

Groin Roll

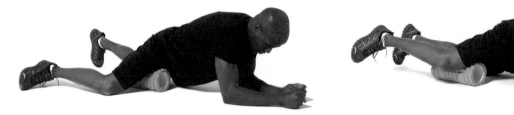

Place the foam roller under your inner thigh, bend your leg and rest on your forearms. Role from the top of your inner thigh to the bottom and back to the starting position. Roll for 2-3 minutes, then switch thighs and repeat.

Calves

Your calf muscles can tighten up from overuse. Playing sports such as basketball, soccer, tennis and football can be hard on your calf muscles. A women's calf muscles can tighten up from wearing high heels. Tight calves can affect your way of walking by limiting the foot and ankle's range of motion and cause heel pain and pain in the arches.

Calf Roll

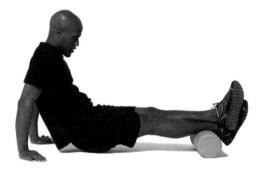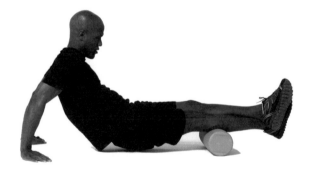

Sit on the floor with the foam roller under your right Achilles tendon and place your left leg on top of your right leg. Place your hands on the floor behind you to support your weight and lift yourself off the floor. Roll from above the Achilles tendon to above your calf and back to the starting position. Roll for 2-3 minutes, then switch calves and repeat.

Foot Arch

There are many factors that can cause arch pain, such as direct trauma, ligament strains, stress fractures and poor alignment. Tight calves can also cause foot pain.

Foot Roll

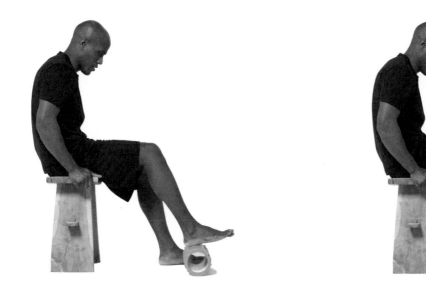

Find something to sit on and place the foam roller under your right heal. Role from the heel through the plantar fascia to the ball of the foot and back to the starting position. Roll for 2-3 minutes, then switch feet and repeat.

Iliotibial Band (IT Band)

If the muscles are tight in your hips or along the side of your leg, you may have IT band syndrome.

Iliotibial Band Roll

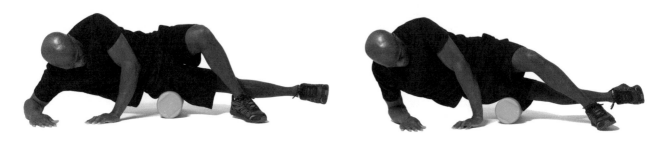

Lie on your right side and place the foam roller under your hip. Place your hands on the floor to support your weight, put your left foot in front of your right leg. Roll from below your hip to above your knee and back to the starting position. Roll for 2-3 minutes, then switch thighs and repeat.

Trap and Shoulder

Our traps can tighten up if we're stressed, from doing too many overhead sports, such as playing tennis, volleyball, baseball and swimming. Your shoulders can become, stiff and sore, if you sit hunched over a computer for a long period of time.

Trap and Shoulder Roll

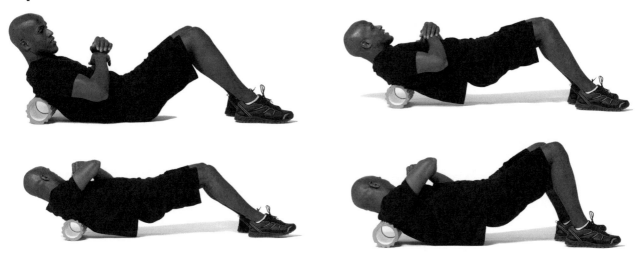

Sit on the floor and place your upper back on the foam roller. Bend your legs, lift your buttocks off the ground and lean your torso to the left. Roll you trap and shoulder back and forth for 2-3 minutes, then switch traps and shoulders and repeat.

Latissimi Dorsi (Lats)

Our lats can tighten up from lifting weights and doing pull ups. Tight lats can cause shoulder mobility to be limited, shoulder pain and rounded shoulders.

Latissimi Dorsi Roll

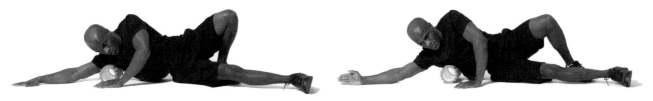

Lie on your right side and place the foam roller under your arm pit. Extend your right arm and place your left hand on the floor to help the motion. Roll from your arm pit to the bottom of your ribs and back to the starting position. Roll for 2-3 minutes, then switch lats and repeat.

Biceps

Our biceps can tighten up from body building and powerlifting. You will not be able to fully extend your arm if your bicep is tight. A tight bicep can lead to shoulder and elbow pain.

Bicep Roll

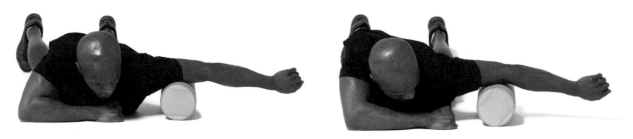

Lie on your stomach and place the foam roller under your left bicep. Rest on your right forearm and roll from your shoulder to the gap between your bicep and forearm and back to the starting position. Roll for 2-3 minutes, then switch biceps and repeat.

Triceps

Our triceps can become weak and tight if we're not doing exercises that targets this muscle. Tight triceps can cause limited mobility at the shoulder or shoulder blade.

Tricep Roll

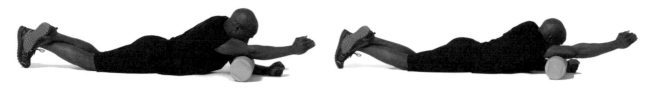

Lie on your stomach and place the foam roller under your right tricep. Rest on your left forearm, roll from your elbow to the end of your tricep and back to the starting position. Make sure you roll the inside and outside of the tricep muscles. Roll for 2-3 minutes, then switch triceps and repeat.

Forearm Muscles

We use our forearm muscles when we open and close our hands, do barbell curls, dumbbell curls, dial a number and when we play the piano. The muscles tighten up because they do a lot of work.

Forearm Roll

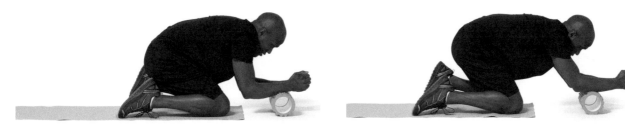

You will need an exercise mat for this exercise. Get down on your knees and place both wrist on the foam roller. Roll from your wrist to your elbows and back to the starting position. Apply pressure with your body and chest while leaning forward. Roll for 2-3 minutes.

Chest

Stand up straight and let your arms hang at your side. If your palms are facing out, your chest muscles are tight and you may have rounded shoulders

Chest Roll

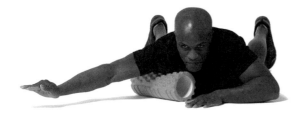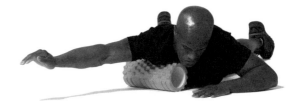

Lie down on your stomach and place the foam roller on an angle under your right pec. Straighten your right arm and rest on your left forearm. Role your pec back and forth for 2-3 minutes, then switch pecs and repeat.

Lacrosse Ball and Exercises

You can use a lacrosse ball for a trigger point massage. What is a trigger point? A trigger point is a sensitive spot in the muscle and connective tissue. Trigger points are caused by muscular overload, repetitive movements, Psychological stress and injury to muscles. Trigger points cause pain and discomfort, weaken muscles, restrict movement and flexibility. When you feel a trigger point, pause and try not to apply pressure. You can also use a lacrosse ball to get to those hard to reach places.

Hamstring Release

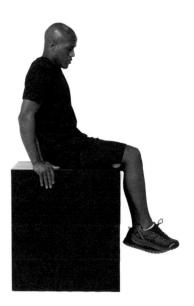 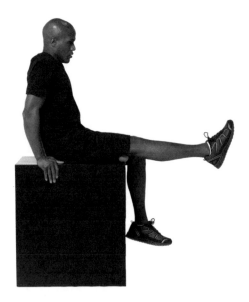

Sit on something hard that will make your feet dangle and place the lacrosse ball under your thigh. Slowly extend your leg and bring it back to the starting position. Do 10 reps, then move the lacrosse ball down your thigh and repeat. Move it down your thigh until you get to your glute, then switch thighs and repeat.

Iliotibial (IT) Band Release

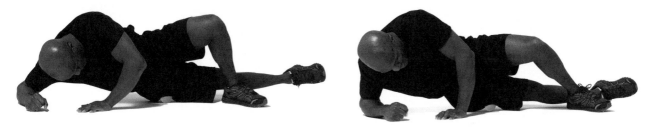

Lie on your right side and place the lacrosse ball below your hip. Rest on your right forearm, place your left hand on the floor, place your left foot in front of your right knee and extend your right leg. Hold that position for 40 seconds to 1 minute, then move the lacrosse ball down your leg and repeat. Move it down your leg until you get to your knee cap, then switch legs and repeat.

Quadricep Release

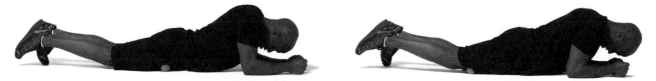

Lie on your stomach with the front of your right thigh on the lacrosse ball and rest on your forearms. Roll from the top of your thigh to your knee cap and back to the starting position. Roll for 2-3 minutes, then switch thighs and repeat.

Calf Release

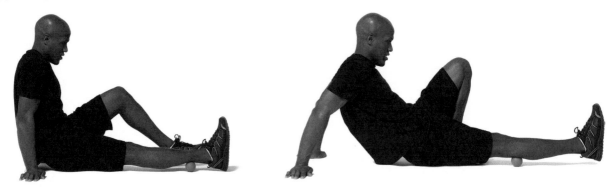

Place your right leg on the lacrosse ball and lift yourself off the ground. Roll your calf from above the Achilles tendon to the top of your calf and back to the starting position. Roll for 2-3 minutes, then switch legs and repeat.

Foot Release

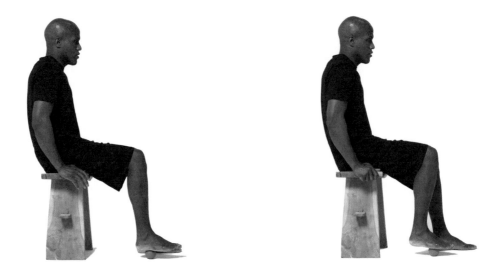

Find something to sit on and place your right foot on the lacrosse ball. Exert pressure on the ball and slowly role the ball from your heel through the plantar fascia to the ball of the foot and back to the starting position. Role your foot for 2-3 minutes, then switch feet and repeat.

Glute Release

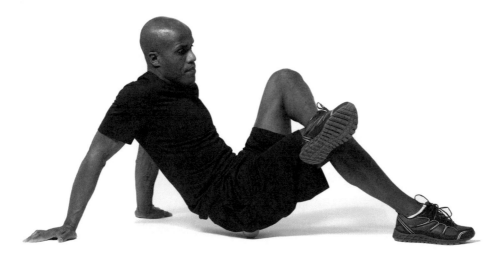

Place your right glute on the ball. Your glute should be a little off to the side. Place your hands on the floor behind you to support your weight, bend your left leg and place it on top of your right leg. Move your glute in a small circular motion for 2-3 minutes, then switch glutes and repeat.

Tensor Fasciae Latae (TFL) Release

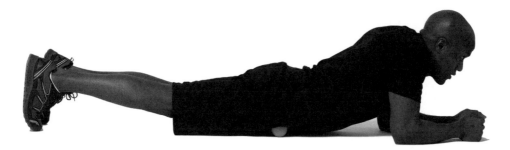

Lie face down, place a lacrosse ball underneath the top of your thigh and rest on your forearms. Hold that position for 1-2 minutes, then switch thighs and repeat.

Spine Release

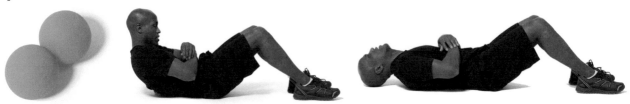

You will need a peanut massager for this exercise. If you don't have one, you can tape two lacrosse balls together. Sit on the ground and place the peanut massager on the ground behind you. Place your mid-to upper back on the peanut massager and center it on your spine. Lay your head on the ground and hold that position for 10 seconds-you should be feeling a stretch. Lift your head and upper back off the ground slowly and go back to the starting position. Do 5-10 repetitions, then move the peanut massager further up the spine and repeat. Move it up the spine until it's centered between your shoulder blades.

Pec Minor and Pec Major Release

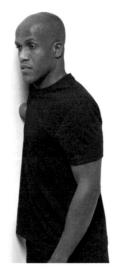

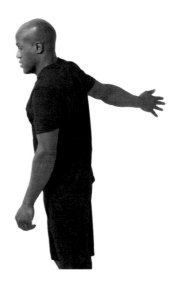

Place the ball on your right pec minor and lean against the wall. Place your right hand against the wall, turn your head to the left and slowly role from your shoulder to the middle of your chest and back to the starting position. Do 20 movements, then switch pecs and repeat.

Resistance Band and Exercises

The resistance band is used in physical therapy, for stretching and strength-training. This tool will help deepen your stretch, stabilize your muscles, improve your balance, prevent injuries and increase your range of motion. The bands come in different sizes, lengths and strengths.

Band Pull Apart

This exercise will strengthen the muscles in your upper back, stabilize the muscles in your shoulder joints and improve your posture.

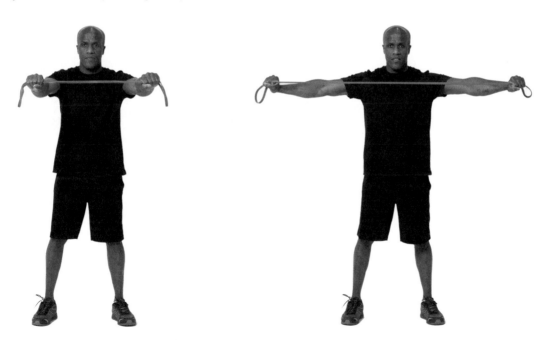

Hold the band with both hands in front of you at shoulder with apart. Your palms should be facing down and your lats pinched back. Stretch your arms to the side and let the band touch your chest. Go back to the starting position and repeat. Do 10-20 repetitions.

X-Band Walk

This exercise targets the core, glutes, hip's and will improve your stability.

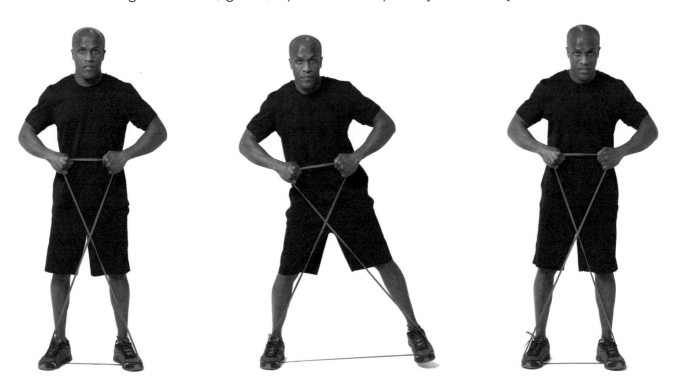

Put the band under your feet and place your feet shoulder width apart. Use your hands and cross the band in front of you. The band should look like an X and held and stretched at mid-torso height. Stand up straight and take ten lateral steps to the right and ten lateral steps to the left. Do 4 sets.

Lateral Band Walk

This exercise will help to improve hip stability, strengthen the hip abductors and increase stability of the knee joint.

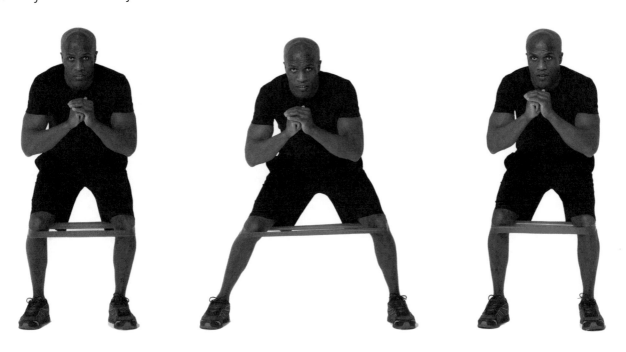

Place a 20 inch band under your knees, Place your feet shoulder-width apart, slightly bend your knees and hips and keep your head and chest up. Take 10 lateral steps to the right and ten lateral steps to the left. Keep your feet shoulder width apart. Do 4 sets.

Banded Hip Distraction

This exercise will help to improve the range of motion of hip abduction and stretch the abductor muscles.

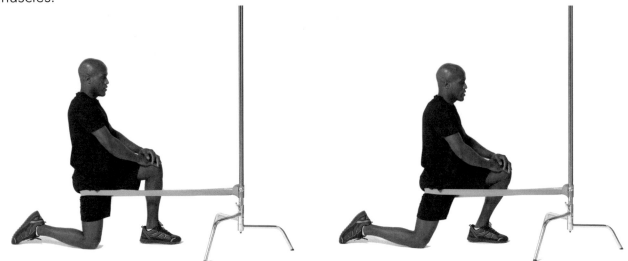

Anchor the band around something that won't move. Hold the band and step into it with your right leg and place it under your glute. Step back as far as you can and kneel on your right knee. Press your hip forward until you feel a good stretch, then go back to the starting position and repeat. Do 10 repetitions, then switch legs and repeat.

Hip Flexor Stretch

This exercise will help to improve the range of motion of hip abduction and stretch the abductor muscles.

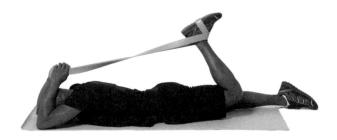 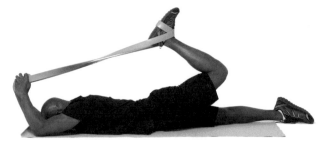

You will need someone to help you with this exercise. Spin the resistance band around your left foot and lie on your stomach. Bend your left leg and get someone to bring the resistance band to your hands. Hold the resistance band and pull it over your back until you feel a good stretch and hold that position for 10-15 seconds, then release and repeat. Do 5 repetitions, then switch feet and repeat.

Hamstring Stretch

If you run, this exercise will help your performance. This exercise will increase the flexibility of the hamstrings, improve your posture, increase blood flow and help prevent injury during a workout.

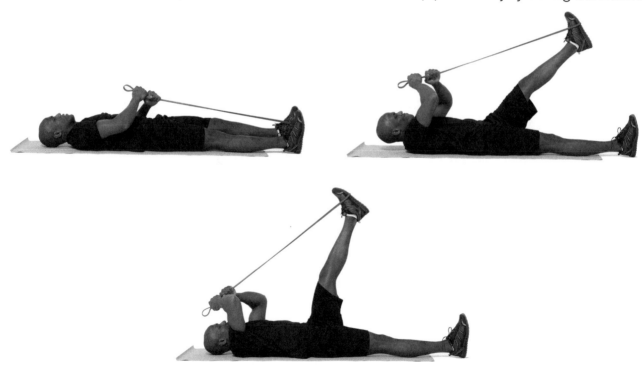

Place the resistance band around your left foot, hold the other end and lie on your back. Keep your right leg straight and pull your left leg towards you. Keep pulling until you feel a good stretch, then hold that position for 5-10 seconds. Release and repeat. Do 5 repetitions, then switch legs.

Groin Stretch

This exercise will improve hip mobility, increase the strength and flexibility of the pelvic floor and the groin.

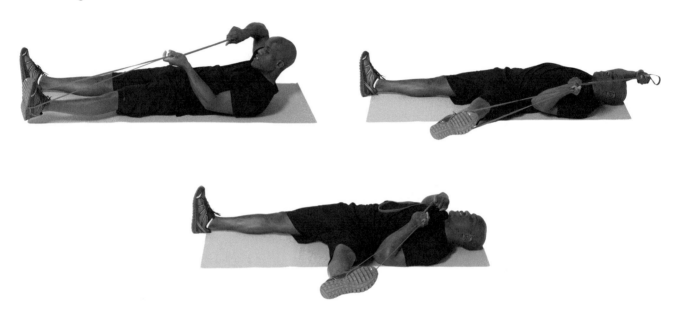

Place the resistance band around your left foot, hold the other end with your right hand, hold the middle with your left hand and lie on your back. Keep your right leg straight and pull your left leg to the left until you get a ninety degree angle. Hold that position for 15-20 seconds, then switch feet and repeat.

Glute Stretch

This exercise will strengthen your legs, improve your posture and increase your blood flow and circulation.

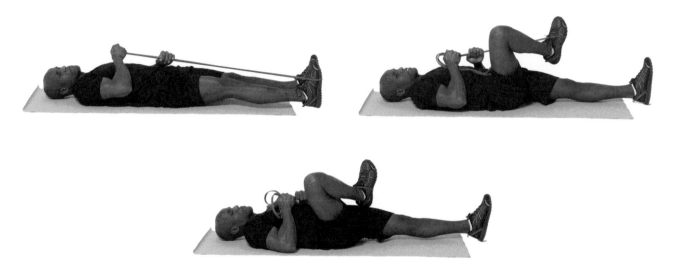

Place the resistance band around your right foot, hold the other end with your right hand and lie on your back. Keep your left leg straight, bend your right leg and pull it towards you. Keep pulling until you feel a good stretch, then hold that position for 10-15 seconds. Switch feet and repeat.

Printed in the United States
By Bookmasters